YOU'RE ALIVE,
But Are You Living?

Raxiel Liz

TABLE OF CONTENTS

PRELUSION

(It's like an intro and stuff!)

Good morning, good afternoon & good night...

I want to start off by saying that there is not an actual right or wrong time to pick up A book and begin reading it. So, whether this is the start of your day, A quick break in the middle or the ending to a hectic one, I want to say thank you! Thank you for picking up a copy and joining me in this mission we call LOVE!

Now... Let's cut the nonsense! As you flip each page, I want you to understand one thing and one thing only. WE ARE NOT IMMORTAL! The Three "L's" (Life, Love and Living) do not wait for anyone. Our worst enemy and best friend is time. (We will get into that later).

I know some of you are reading this saying "Isn't Life and Living the same thing?" NOOOO!!! It is not the same thing! "Life" is what is around you, People, your atmosphere, your job etc.... Things that you have no control of and will continue existing with or without you. Now "Living" is how you choose to interact (Live) in that life.

Sir Thomas Browne said: "We are living on borrowed time"

The Bible stated: **Proverbs 27:1** Do not boast about tomorrow, for you do not know what a day may bring.

Estrella Liz Said: "Life is one big joke... Waiting to be laughed at"

That last quote was from my mother (R.I.P.)

Now... where does "Love" fall in all of this? DEAD

SMACK

IN THE MIDDLE!

Remember... You are not **Immortal!**

Every second, minute, hour, day, month, and year! LOVE IT!

CHAPTER 1

THE KICK IN THE NUTS TRUTH

(OR VAGINA YOU KNOW WHAT I MEAN)

THE KICK IN THE NUTS TRUTH

The day you are born... Everybody loves you. I mean why the hell not; everyone loves babies right? You are a blessing, a gift or maybe someone's life changing experience. Either way you look at it, babies always bring out another side of people. The love for a baby has made people change their entire outlook on life. (Now you do have the occasional Buttholes who do cruel things to infants and kids but, we are not going to get into that today.) Back to my point everyone loves you right? You are the baby, you meet mom and dad for the first time, you get taken to your new home maybe meet the cat or dog, maybe even both. You may or may not have an older brother or sister, and until you become a teenager everything is just about handed to you as much as possible. YOU ARE THE PRINCE/PRINCESS!

Ok here comes the kick! You are a teenager now... 13 going on no one understands me!

SIDE NOTE: *I am aware that there may be a few that read this part of the book and cannot relate... Some parents get lucky with some of us and have teenagers that don't think the entire world is against them and that no one understands them because they have life all figured out!*

Now that we got that nonsense out the way... Like I was saying, you are a teenager now and life can be tricky. You are making some decisions of your own and allowed to do certain things you weren't able to do before. Life begins to open in directions that should come with an instruction manual. This is the part of life I call the free fall. See as a teen the universe tends to test us in so many ways. A lot of us do not realize that A large portion of our pain, guilt, frustration, and other negative energies is carried over from our teenage years to adulthood. We free fall through so many different obstacles in life as a teen and the emergency string to open the parachute is nowhere in sight!

Let me be transparent with you for a minute... My brother was murdered in front of me at the age of 14. We were all in a car driving back from the movie theater in New York. The time was about 12:30 AM and we arrived at the corner of 167 street Findlay avenue in the Bronx. There were, if I recall correctly, 6 of us in the car. I was sitting on my brother's lap in the back seat because I couldn't fit. His friend noticed a man and woman arguing by the corner store. The guy seemed to be putting his hands on the woman and hurting her. My brothers friend asked if everything was ok to the woman. That is when we all realized that this man was not all there. We believe he was high on something and drunk. In a panic and fear that we were going to do something to him and defend the woman, he pulled out a gun. This was my first official descend

into my "Free fall". The man starts shooting at the car and my brother's friend quickly got back in and drove off! He drove with his head down, so we bumped and damaged a few other cars on the way down the hill trying to avoid the gun fire. I yelled to my brother "Keep your head down", that was when I realized what happened… He was already shot and dead. His blood was gushing from the side of his head onto my neck and shoulders. In a panic I yelled "Please stop the car I believe he has been shot!" I get out of the car and tried to pull his nonresponsive body out. Everyone surrounded me, there was so much screaming and yelling I could not focus and one of his friends picked me up and put me back in the car. We zoomed to the hospital where he was pronounced dead at around 2:30 AM.

Free falling deeper and deeper in seconds…. All I could think was when will I wake up! Please God let this be a nightmare that I am going to snap out of in a second. No, it was real, and it was getting worst by the minute. One of the most painful things I ever had to do in my life was call my mother and tell her the horrible event that took place that night.

Ok… Now that I have expressed and given some insight on some of my beginnings let's get back on track. Let us fast forward to adult hood. As I said earlier, we carry a lot of luggage into our adult lives. I wanted to be transparent to show that what I write and explain is real. I am not here writing and trying to preach on subjects I have no idea about. I am not here to speak on topics that I have studied and have not gone through. I am not a therapist (Even though everyone says I need to be). The subjects we will touch on together are from experience.

"The kick in the nuts" about life is that it does not give a freak about your opinion. Now do not get me wrong, life is an amazing journey filled with beautiful places, people, and experiences but, that's just it! For every up there is a down... It is the unfair exchange of the universe. Life is not fair and we as people shouldn't be scared! With all the hurdles we must jump and sometimes duck down and crawl under, we must stay diligent! We must keep going.... We must LOVE IT! Playing a game is not fun if it doesn't challenge you. If it were an easy game, you would complete it and get bored of it quickly. That is why success in life feels good, acing a test that you studied hard for or over coming something that has scared you for a long time feels amazing once you reach the top. Now once you've reached the top get ready... Life is standing there with a sword made of fire riding a pink unicorn!

I promise it will all make sense.

CHAPTER 2

BEST FRIEND &
WORST ENEMY

(Depending on how you look at it… They're the same)

BEST FRIEND AND WORST ENEMY

Procrastination

Hesitation

Vacillation…

Three words that are the best friend to your enemy. You can add the word "Fear" in the mix to make a nice disaster "I'm never going to get anything done" soup! The process of creating is an amazing one! It doesn't matter if you are an artist, teacher, stylist etc.… Whatever your craft, the worst thing you can do is any of these three. P.H.V. (Procrastination, Hesitation & Vacillation) are dream killers, light diminishers and the vanquishers of hope!

*Some may say that P.H.V. are all three in the same. I beg to differ.
Let us break the three down and see how they affect us daily.*

Procrastination: Being an asshole with yourself and giving yourself a hundred reasons why you don't just start!

Hesitation: Being a sissy and acting like there is something holding you back once you get to the starting point.

Vacillation: Not being able to make a freaking decision!

Each different but, all three lead to the same outcome... Not getting anything done! As people we at times fear the subject of choice. It's easy to sit back and look at someone else and make a decision for them but, when it comes to our-selves there is a huge invisible wall. That wall is called Fear. This all goes back to chapter one where we covered "if it were easy it wouldn't be entertaining or satisfying". When it comes to creating you must take risks. You cannot stand there and P.H.V. your way through it! Stop being a sucker about it! It's better to fail and learn from your failure rather than not try at all and never know what the outcome could have been. Then, you are haunted with the self-doubt and curiosity of what could have been and never find out!

Motivated by the stand still moment... That is something I used to suffer from, which falls in with Procrastination. Something I struggled with in a major way. You ever notice when things are going ok or running smoothly your dreams and ambitions don't attack the back of your heart, mind, body, and soul? Then suddenly the day comes when you are frustrated, agitated at work, or just plain and simple mad at the world you start saying things to yourself.

I need to do this...

I need to finish that...

I need to find a way out of this!

That becomes your thought process. That is when you allow yourself to be motivated by the stand still moments. The moments when your life feels like it's going nowhere, and life is riding by with that sword made of fire riding that pink unicorn looking down at you tapping it's watch! I repeat this again and I am sure I will some more throughout this book... WE ARE NOT IMMORTAL!!!

If you haven't caught on yet, the subject we have been referring to in this chapter is "Time"... Time can be your worst enemy but, at the same time (pun intended) it can be your best friend! Even though when it comes to time, we should never P.H.V. but, at the same time we must know when to take our time. To some this may be confusing, and I understand why. Don't get all frantic and jump out the window just yet calm, your ass down and let me explain. Granted you should never P.H.V. but, Patience, Pacing and prepping are three ways to utilize your time. Again, the sole purpose of this journey is to understand LOVE. Although time can be our enemy, it can also become a friend we can love and cherish!

Patience: The opposite of Procrastination...
Consider it being smart while waiting.

Pacing: Knowing when to move and not
rush it. Think like a chess player.

Prepping: Staying ready so you don't have to get ready!

P.P.P. (Patience, Pacing & Prepping) is the art of taking your enemy (Time) and turning it into your biggest ally. Basically, taking time and calmly making it your own! We cannot control time but, we can flow with it and not allow it to leave us behind. Remember that we cannot get time back nor can we beat time in a race… You must move with it, you must understand your time frame and know when to strike, when to move, and when to stand still and wait.

Identify your enemy = P.H.V.

Utilize your allies = P.P.P.

Next time you see life on that unicorn with the burning sword stand strong, be patient, and as soon as life swoops down to try and strike you, you can dodge it's attack…. piss on its fire sword… extinguish the flame…. and look back at it and say… You don't want no smoke bitch!

Time! -Find your niche… Understand it and make it work for you not against you- We don't have 99 lives, we can't Up, up, down, down, left, right, left, right, A, B, Start our way through this. (That was for my gamers if you didn't understand that ask a true gamer). We must deal with it; we must live with it and most of all… It will better benefit you if you

···

LOVE IT!

Time waits for no one, but everyone is trying to make or find time! WTF?

CHAPTER 3

SHE HATES IT TODAY

(you're in trouble now!)

SHE HATES IT TODAY

They say life's a "B" and then you die... hmm?

I need someone to explain this one to me. So, your trying to tell me because the universe wasn't feeling it, I have to suffer? F.O.H. (Freak Outta Here). Ok let us get serious, let me break down what I am trying to say here, She Hates It Today.

You wake up and get ready for a regular day. Brush your teeth, get dressed, make your coffee, and head out the door. So far so good... You get in your car and drive off. Here comes that Pink Unicorn and flaming sword! You get on the main street only to hit traffic! You haven't even been driving for 5 minutes and already your entire day is delayed! Now you are stuck in traffic with nothing to do but, listen to the radio. You choose talk radio (Why I don't know it's what we do, we suffer to listen to other people suffer so we all freaking suffering!) The podcast is covering a story about something terrible that happen last night. So now you are stuck in traffic and listening to bad news going on around the world. You notice that the traffic is thicker than you expected so you call your job and tell them you are going to be late. Your boss who is always a stressed-out butthole gives you nonsense about a situation you cannot control (Traffic). 45 minutes to an hour later you finally get to work, and everyone is complaining! The workload is over the top and unfair to the staff. Co-workers are looking at you like you intended to be late on purpose. Like you just knew that today would be the day to have a traffic jam and delay your entire day out of sheer asshole-ism! It's a long day, your boss is stressed, so he takes it out on you! On your lunch break your favorite restaurant was burned down because the owner was cheating on his wife and she retaliated by burning down his establishment! You are forced to eat at a fast food place that has nasty food and bad service... Let's fast forward the day, shall we? You finally make it back home from a crappy day, you take a shower, decompress, watch a little tv and have a drink... The day is over.

It is safe to say that this was a bad day, right? But ask yourself this... Who was it a bad day for? You or them? OR!!!!!!!!!!!!! The universe? Look up, YUP! Pink Unicorn, Yup Flaming sword!

The part we are missing is that we (You) didn't necessarily have a bad day. Nothing wrong or bad happen to you. Yes, there was traffic, yes you got to work late and yes people were complaining and complaining all day but, honestly was it really that bad when you look back at it?

OK let's look at the facts! Traffic jams are common and if you went through one every day at the same time then that is your own fault for not realizing that you need to leave the house earlier.

Take that coffee to go! But, in this case that wasn't the issue was it? You know the time you should leave your house, you have been doing this for a while so it's safe to say that this particular day something went wrong on the road which caused everything to be backed up. Pay attention! Nothing you did caused this. You got to work late and because your idiot manager was stressed out like they always are (because they only do the same freaking job every single mother freaking day and still somehow drop the ball daily and get stressed out every single minute of the day all due to their bad time management skills!) It's safe to say you probably feel you can do your bosses job better than his/her stupid self! Co-workers are upset blah blah lick my balls blah!

Breathe...

Take a second...

Observe your surroundings...

You didn't have a bad day... The universe had a bad day (Or caused one) Mother earth wasn't feeling it today! S.H.I.T. (She Hates It Today). We as people need to understand that we are all in this together and sometimes our surroundings can cause us to be taken off course. It's the obstacles of life. Again, if you haven't already understood my point... You didn't have a bad day, the universe did. The people around you did, your dumb boss did, your co-workers did, the store owner who cheated on his wife and got his place burned down did! NOT YOU!!! We live on this beautiful planet and others do to. It spins but, not around us. Everyone is not in this world with you, you are in this world with them. You cannot let things that are out of your control bother you. Yes, I know it can be hard at times but, it's a muscle you have to work on and give it it's daily exercise to master. If you look back, everything is ok. You didn't lose your job, your car works, and you are ok.

I would never encourage feeling good over someone else's

pain and suffering but, at the same time, you must learn how to brush things off and realize the blessings, gifts or luck (Which ever floats your boat) you have. We live in a world where any moment something can go wrong, and that wrong is completely out of our control. That is where P.P.P. (Patience, Pacing and Prepping) come back into play. If the world around you (Life = Pink Unicorn & Flaming sword) is having a bad day, you need to learn how to separate yourself from it and dodge the obstacles it leaves behind.

You ever seen someone having a bad day. They are expressing their anger; their body language just screams "I'm going to kill someone or myself today"! It is obvious you need to leave this person alone. Then you or someone else didn't take heed of the signs the universe was putting in front of you and accidently interact with this individual and BOOM! You are in a full-blown argument with a complete stranger! Maybe even a fight! This is technically your fault. You noticed the "S.H.I.T." You realized that life is a pain and today! Life wasn't messing around and was shaking the building. You just ended up staring down the unicorn's butt crack! But, instead of noticing the smell of ass, peanuts and chopped onion coming out of the unicorn's pie hole you recklessly inserted your head inside and got crapped on! Who's fault is that? Life is like a game and you only have one life and a limited amount of health. Now you can increase the health and longevity of that one life but, you cannot make it last forever... WE ARE NOT IMMORTAL! In a racing game when you are driving the car 100 M.P.H. (Miles per hours) you don't just go straight and not pay attention. Many different things will happen while playing that game. You will obviously crash, flip your car 52 times, hit someone or go flying out the windshield face first with the wind blowing your face and mouth back exposing all your teeth as you collide teeth first into a brick wall! THAT IS LIFE!!! When you are sleep, you are going about 15 M.P.H. I say that because even in your sleep something can go wrong with you or around you. Now when you wake up and put your crusty feet on the ground, you are going about 32 M.P.H. But, when you step out your house you go from 32 to 180 instantly, with no breaks and a cinder block strapped to your foot, duck tapped and glued to the peddle plus the breaks are nowhere to be found!

All in all, you need to acknowledge the "L's" and utilize the middle mostly!

1: Life = The Individual holding that flaming sword on a Pink Unicorn!

2: Love = Just shut up and Love! It is not going anywhere. Enjoy the ride.

3: Living = You are in this sissy for the long run, so live it to the fullest! Don't just cry and die!

A famous artist once said "Everybody dies but, not everybody lives"

Don't let that be you.

Someone once said "Life's a "B" and then you die!"... So does the "B" lives forever?

CHAPTER 4

FIST FIGHTING
WITH GHOST

(PLACE YOUR BETS)

FIST FIGHTING WITH GHOSTS

A sensitive topic even for me but, still must be prepped up, cooked, eaten and pooped out! So, knuckle up!

Let me start off by asking do you walk backwards? When you drive do you only use your rear-view mirror? Or better yet... When you go to the bathroom to poop out last night's dinner... Do you stick your hands in the toilet and eat what you crapped out to taste how good the food from last night was? Of course not., If you are looking at the page as you read this and making a "That was nasty face" then you are in need of this chapter! If you read this and smiled or giggled or better yet sitting in a public place and laughed out loud, looked around and realized you look crazy to others, then you are on the right track!

Unicorns... "Ahem" excuse me I mean "Life" doesn't understand the concept of "Do overs, Rewind or Pause". Once an event takes place it's on and popping and there is no turning back! I agree it freaking sucks on a non-magnanimous level! Unicorns

(Life) do not look back and do not feel guilt, pain, or remorse. This is why the phrase "Unicorn" (Life) is used this way in this book... "Tunnel vision". You ever watch a horse race? What is the horse trained to do... Run but, not only run... Run in one direction and one mission! That mission is forward! Not only is it trained to run forward they make sure it is not distracted by adding blinders on the side of each eye. That is life, life is meant to keep going with no questions asked! Now life is a special gift! Therefore, it cannot just be a horse... It is a Unicorn with its rider wielding a sword ingulfed in fire!

Now let's get to you fist fighting these ghost and what life and unicorns have to do with that! Back to the gamers... You ever played a game and as you are playing you realized you missed something but, the game does not let you go back to get it. You missed it tough luck! Yup! That is life... We don't get do overs; we don't get "Oh snap my bad I'll do it better next time". Once it's done it's done! Now let's get deep...

Deep...

DEEP!!!

When you break up with someone, when you lose something, or better yet when your dog/cat dies or you lose a loved one! In my case like I said in the 1st chapter, I lost my Mom to Cancer, my brother was killed in front of me and my dad won the lottery and was murdered for the ticket. You know what all three of those have in common? No rewind button, no way to pause it and no matter how much I "Fist Fight with These Ghost" they are not coming back!

Divorced, can't see your kids, and you have to go through 100 court meetings to convince the masses that you are sane enough to see your kid.... yeah... No going back and fixing that. Your boyfriend/husband or girlfriend/wife cheated on you with your best friend... yeah... No going back and fixing that! Or better yet you lose your mom or dad... That's not even a go back and fix situation because you had no control over that whatsoever, but again can't change it! It is what it is! Now with that being said, I am not saying chuck it to the wind, man up and forget about it! No! We need to realize one thing while we are going through the pain... We cannot rewind time, so crying and hoping you will wake up from your nightmare is not going to happen. Crying is good for the soul, we as people must cry and let out that pain and hurt! What is not good for the soul is False hope, False Thoughts, and False perception. There is nothing worse than getting to the end of a road of pain and realizing that your entire mission was in vein! It's like... What the hell!

It's ok to remember and reminisces but, it's poison to dwell on past events. These Unicorns don't give a crap! By the time you even begin to kind of cope with the pain you have been bamboozled with they already forgot who you are! They forgot what they did, they forgot they even passed by your neighborhood! Regret is a pill that if swallowed it's almost impossible to throw back up! Regret is a poison that darkens the soul and creates demons. Along with regret comes pain, self-hate & more. Ghost (Our emotions and thoughts) haunt us, leaving us punching the air! (Fist fighting with ghost).

Death isn't the only form of a ghost... Doubt, neglect and the occasional "Could've, would've, should've are extreme ghost that haunt the soul and mind. When Unicorns do their thing (When life takes its course) we are not in control, we are all along for the ride. We inflict most of our decisions on ourselves on some stupid dumb stuff. How many of us have cheated raise your hand? If you raised your hand while reading this book you are fucking crazy and you need to film yourself doing it or take a picture and send it to me on Instagram @raxiel_liz because I would love to see that! I'm kidding, if you raised your hand or raised your hand in your mind then you have been a victim of the "Could've, would've, should've situation. It's like you start thinking back to yourself and saying, "What the hell was I thinking, why did I do that?" Was it worth it?.... GHOST! You are haunted by the skeletons in your closet you filthy animal. Who keeps dirty old bones in their closet?

Ok let's put all these dead bodies, regrets and stupid decisions in a pile and analyze this shall we? When we lose someone we love 9 out of 10 times it's due to a situation we couldn't control. Random crap like "cancer, brain aneurysm, or killed" no matter how you cut it at the end, it's not your fault... But some of us love to act like it was. We say things like "I wish I said this while they were alive, I wish I did that while they were alive, and I wish they were here now so I can blah blah blah! I feel you and I agree. I feel the same way! You know how many times I wish my mother was here to celebrate my accomplishments, you know how many times I wish I got shot instead of my brother but, what would it matter because if it was me that got shot, it might have been him writing this book wishing he got shot instead of me! (See how that works). The Unicorns are not fair... The Unicorns don't sit back and take a second to adjust all of the possible outcomes. They just act!

Life docs not have to be as complicated as we make it. Too many of us complain, cry, and wish, then by the time they decide to get over it or adjust they look back and they are 50 years old! Let go... Forgive yourself and others... But when it comes to others never forget. If you forget you allow yourself to get jerked all over again in a greater way! Plus, the fact that your butt has been torn before it is harder to heal the 2nd time around. Move forward, look at yourself in the mirror and face fear head on! You only live once and in some cases it's not for that long of a time frame, take it from the people we have lost. Use it, embrace it, allow it to make you stronger. Take those scars and turn them into alligator skin!

A secret about people... They get tired of being supportive to a negative broken cause. Not everyone but, the ones we need the most are the ones who disappear 1st! (Not all the time but, you get my drift). Even if you disagree and you just happen to be one of those people who has not been let down by others... Consider yourself lucky and blessed but, at the same time don't you want to be strong for yourself, for them, for the next time the Unicorn decides to rear it's beautiful face? Learn from pain... Be real with pain... Understand your pain!!! Don't allow the pain to knock you down, knock the pain out of your system.

You ever been made fun of or witness someone being made fun of? You ever notice that if the person being attacked isn't fazed by it the person doing the attacking stops? It's not funny unless the person being attack shows some kind of emotional disturbance. Same thing with pain. The more realistic you are with yourself and your pain, the easier it is to handle it. Not necessarily get over the pain but, know how to handle the pain. Too many times dwelling in their past pain can break a person, and that individual doesn't know they have been shattered into tiny pieces.

Your past is the past, the present is currently happening, and your future will pass you by if you are not paying attention because your devoting to much attention to the past. Imagine your future becoming your past because in the present you only focused on the past? It's an unfair game called Life and we entered our quarters, pressed start, selected a character, and didn't realize we only have one life! So, you can hate it and live unhappy because the unicorns didn't answer your calling... Or enjoy the ride grab the unicorn by the balls and Don't just be Alive, LIVE!

Imagine watching a movie based on your life?

How many stars would you rate it and would you enjoy the movie?

Explore, be strong and embrace your past and pain and live!

Don't worry, when you die your past and the dead will be there waiting for you.

You can't go back to the past... But your past can come back to bite you in the BUTT!

CHAPTER 5

PISSING ON
YOUR HEART

(RELATIONSHIP GOALS)

PISSING ON YOUR HEART

Oh oh... This is a sensitive tricky don't let it slip into my butt subject. (Not that anything is wrong with that if that is what you're into cool). Relationships!...... It's funny because 9 out of 10 times people don't know what they want out of them. When asked people say funny and silly things like, "I want someone smart and pretty, sexy but, casual serious but, has a sense of humor, crazy but, not insane!" Okay... So, you want a Bi-polar, uncertain, insecure, smart ass with an endless pointless faucet of social media I read it online knowledge individual that tells you they love you every other Sunday?

Ask yourself this... Did you screen your friends before you

met them? It's ironic that no matter what you are (Male/Female) We tend to do the same shit! We always look for someone as if we are ordering a cup of coffee.

"Hello Yes, can I have a medium coffee, Splenda with a little bit of brown sugar, low fat milk, whip cream, 2 shots of expresso but, please make the coffee a light roast with a smooth blend but bold. Also, can I have a splash of coconut but, not from concentrated... oh yeah and a nonfat soymilk muffin".

This is either you or you definitely know the type! The crazy part is why we as individuals don't use the same tactics we use when meeting new friends, when we are trying to meet a potential partner? That tactic and skill is called "BE YOUR FREAKING SELF!" When you met your best friend or any friend that you consider great! You weren't putting on a show, you weren't trying to be cool and impress them. You were just being you and if they vibe with that then cool if they didn't, get the hell out of my face right!?

The same skills and tactics should always be used when meeting someone you like for a partner etc.... Don't force it, if it happens it happens. A simple hello and how are you goes a long way. If you are at a bar and you meet a person do not be a cocky penis (That's a penis, penis!) and try to impress the person. Don't follow the unwritten rules of engagement that were created by a unknow idiot years ago when the time frame was horse and carriage. Especially men, we love to act like we are some kind of supernatural gentleman that fell from the heavens and all of a sudden, we are cool, smooth, spit fire out your mouth too! If that is not who you are then don't pretend to be that guy when you meet someone.

Let me explain a major mistake Men and Women make

when meeting someone. They lie... What I mean by that 9 out of 10 times, as much as we want to be sincere, we talk to a certain person based off looks 1st. I mean it's ok, it's the first thing we see right? Their face, body, what they are wearing, how they look etc. As much as we hate to admit it we are judging the person to see if they are worth walking up to and starting a conversation with. I know someone is reading this saying I don't do that, I search for their energy in the air, I wait for the universe to connect us and slide me over with an avocado filled with strawberries. Please SHUT THE HELL UP AND SKIP TO THE NEXT CHAPTER IF YOU MUST!

Let us be real... There is nothing wrong with wanting to speak with someone you find attractive. The problem starts when you or that person begin to act like someone you are not. When you go out on a date, if you are not the (put your jacket over a puddle type) then why the hell would you do that? What puddle in history have you seen that he/she couldn't jump over or walk around? Plus, in my opinion that person should take into consideration that if you wore that jacket to meet them, then that was a firm selection and you really like that jacket... Why would they want you to intentionally mess it up? Just mean! All in all, when meeting someone just be your freaking self! If they do not like that then it's not meant to be.

Too many times people are in relationships and everything is going pretty good for about a year or two, then they move in together and all hell breaks loose. You start to see who the person really is. How messy they are, how they are at home, what habits do they have etc... Word to the wise, if you can't act the same way you act around your friends with your partner... Then it's most likely not going to work! Your partner is supposed to be your friend, YOUR BEST FRIEND DUMMY! If you can't talk to them in the same manner, laugh about the same things, joke, cry, enjoy the same things you do with your friends, I bet there will be a stopping point in the relationship! I know someone is reading this like "You don't know shit" ....that's because YOUR relationship is in the shit spot. Let's move on...

Learn this, if you don't shut the hell up and love yourself then don't expect to succeed in loving someone else. Honesty is the best policy when it comes to your heart! The divorce rate in the United States is so high that marriage now a days is a joke. The reason is people are marrying who they like, not who they genuinely love! Your partner should be your best freaking friend and I mean best friend. For example, if your boys say let's have a guy's night out and you can't bring your partner, you kind of wouldn't want to go and vice versa for the ladies. How many times have you had a guy's/lady's night out and it seems like a relief! If that is the case something is wrong, especially if you and your friends are bad mouthing each other's partner. You got the game messed up!

You are who you are and that cannot change. If it does, you're probably going to be an unhappy son of a B..... I know too many people in relationships who have lost themselves and who they are years ago! Relationship goals should be fun, success, and longevity. Not frustration, anger and empty pockets! Speaking of broke, anyone who is in a relationship with money problems that fight due to money issues, do yourself the favor and break up today! You guys are not real! Forget you, forget him and forget her! True love and happiness are not measured in wealth and material things. It's funny how people fight and argue over issues like money. If they took all that energy and channeled it into their finances, ideas, and game plan for each other maybe they can get out of their financial situation TOGETHER! Together they can become a King and Queen. The days that the guy pays all of the bills are over! Who the hell made that stupid rule anyway? Now... If you as the guy want to do that, by all means, knock yourself out but, how could you call your relationship a team or goals when you have different pockets? You have different agendas when it comes to that? How could you build an empire separately? Don't lie to yourselves, at the end it's all insecurity, greed, and mistrust! Everyone knows if you want to test a friendship or relationship just throw money in the mix!

Let's talk Sex, the nitty gritty, bumping uglies, making love, freaking or as I like to call it "Throwing Trash"! A relationship does not succeed without what?

COMMUNICATION!!!!!!!!!!!!!!!!!!!!!!!

Talking, Understanding, reaching agreements, sharing, trust, honor, honesty, respect and here it comes... Throwing Trash (Remember I said that meant sex). In a relationship Throwing trash is up there with finances. It's something that you both need and have to be open and honest about! Plus, it needs to happen. In a relationship there is no such thing as too soon! It's either just right or not! If you like or love the person truly... Then what is the problem? Especially if you have been in a relationship with them for years. How long you chose to wait before throwing trash with someone after you meet them is up to you. But, let me tell you this, you can wait 1 day, or you can wait 1 year the outcome most likely will be the same. If you guys are truly into each other and being honest, then it will turn out ok. If there is fakeness involved, distrust or someone is not being real and honest, trust that no matter how long it takes, after it happens it will crumble the same way it would of if it happened earlier. I mean, might as well get it out the way and see what happens!

Don't get me wrong, I am not saying go out a sleep with everyone or anyone. Please do not take it like that (if you did, you must have not been reading the pages correctly). There is no reading between the lines here. This is as raw and uncut as it can get. You own your life, your world, your wellbeing. Ask yourself where did the instruction manual come from? Who set these ideas, these stats, these ridiculous steps into how to go about a relationship? Everyone is different, everyone doesn't function the same therefore, the situation should be based off of your gut feeling and instincts. How many people you know go about their relationships the way we have been programmed to and it ends in chaos? You know what else is programmed into people as well? The way they rain chaos after the marriage or relationship doesn't work.

It's a kind of a crazy shame that there are ads and banners for lawyers waiting for us to break up and fight! All that is programmed into us the same way some of the silly steps are. Be real with yourself, only you can look after you. Here we go again with the P.H.V and not the P.P.P. Most people go through about 4 to 5 relationships before they meet someone they stay with and have longevity with. Ever wonder why? Sometimes it's luck, sometimes it's because they went the (let's be real) route and sometimes it's because they finally developed thick skin, are not taking any crap, and approached the situation in a "this is me take it or leave it or forget you" attitude. THEY WERE REAL. They weren't trying to play princess or prince; they weren't trying to act like a baller or the gentlemen they are not. She wasn't acting like she is the most innocent female on the planet, he/she put their penis and breast on the table along with the truth and said, "this is me, this is what I want and this is what I got, so what thehell is up you in or out?"

It's a way of life Boy meets girl, girl likes boy.
It's all a risk no matter how you approach it.

This is the game of life... Enjoy the game and play it wisely.

You have to play so just LOVE it.

A broken heart doesn't require surgery.

CHAPTER 6

SQUARE DANCING IN A CIRCLE

(IF YOU DON'T FIT IN STAND OUT!)

SQUARE DANCING IN A CIRCLE

As people, we seek a few basic things out of others, but one that has become a huge problem in today's society is "Acceptance". It is pretty funny if you think about it. People want to be themselves and be original but, feel bad when they're not accepted into a trend or click of some kind. This is a subject that has damaged the world in many ways. Especially with social media and other platforms. Being accepted has become a part of people's well-being and mental stability. Well, we as people need to learn to practice the "Forget em" treatment. They don't like you? "Forget em"... They don't think your cool enough? "Forget em" Oh, they feel like they are better than you? "Fotget em"

Forget em'

FORGET EM'!!!!!!!!!!!!

F

O

R

G

E

T

FORGET   E M'

(Let's talk about it)

To get the record straight yes, we all know it sucks when people don't accept you for who you are. Yes, we can all agree on that! On the flip side, there is nothing more satisfying than being accepted for who you are! To tell you the truth, people AIN'T nothing or they are a PIECE of crap or... they think they're THE best! (Same difference) With all that crap flying around you as an individual need to not GIVE a crap! You know why the world seems bright at times and it seems like the sun is out even though you don't see it at the moment? It's because that light you are seeing causing the day to appear bright and shiny isn't the sun... No... That light belongs to the fire that is attached to that sword being held by that person riding the pink Unicorn (Life). Life goes on and it does not care if you do or don't. Same thing with those that don't accept you for who you are.

If you eat a piece of chicken that looks good and smells good but, when you finally take a bite and the chicken taste like racoon nuts sautéed in hot wolf knuckles... What do you do?

A. Do you keep eating it because it looked good and smelled good?

B. Do you keep chewing it because you want it to taste good?

C. Do you spit it out and sucker punch the cook?

If you chose "C" then you are a mean rude person, just because you don't like something doesn't mean you slap the freaking cook but, you are on the right track! You are right, you spit it out! No one wants to eat something that taste bad to them. Not only that, if you didn't like it, I am sure you wouldn't come back the next day to the same place and order the same nasty dish, would you? No... not at all why would you?

Here is another scenario before we continue... have you ever ate poop? Like actual poop, dung, crap, caca, mierlda, doodoo, booboo? Well have you? Why not? I am sure no one reading this has! Reason being is because we already know it's something we are not going to like, we don't need to go outside and walk our dog, pick up their poop, and eat it to know we are not going to enjoy it. If you ate a nice juicy steak, seasoned to the core, nice bed of rice and beans or whatever you consider to be your favorite plate... after you poop it out... do you eat it because you know that even though it's shit, you know deep inside it's actually your favorite dish just mushed up in to what is now shit! No? Why not? BECAUSE IT'S SHIT AND WE KNOW WE DON'T LIKE IT!!!!

Ok back on topic (Not that we ever left) We know we don't eat poop... So why do we want poop in our lives? Remember in high school the "cool kids"? Why were they cool and who were they cool to? If the cool kids don't accept you because you are not cool enough, you as an individual need to understand that it isn't that you are not cool, it's that you are not their cup of tea and they are not yours. Let's say you are a Gamer; you love video games and comic books etc.... If you did hang out with the cool kids, there is a big possibility that they are not into that. They might be into typical materialistic things like sports, cars, cheer leading, make up (Depending on the gender) and you are not! So, are you not cool to them or are they not cool to you? Besides, who told you they were cool? If no one else was riding them and no one in the building was paying them any mind, would you even acknowledge them? Would you even know they were there? Or, would they seem invisible how you feel you appear to them?

The world around us was damaged before social media; social media just destroyed it, and we destroyed social media! Now don't get it wrong, social media has helped the world in many wonderful ways (you probably wouldn't be reading this book if you didn't find it on social media) but, the point I'm trying to make is we allow the world around us to influence our train of thought. When you are at home and pick up on things you like during your own time. You picked up what caught your interest. It could have been from what we said earlier comics, video games, sports, cars, modeling, fashion, etc... Male or female, it doesn't matter what it was/is that you took interest in. The point here is why do you want to be accepted in a crowd that does not do or like the same things as you?

-Contradiction-

With that being said, we also have to be real with ourselves and take into consideration, that just because someone doesn't like what you like does not mean you cannot be friends with them or connect in some way. It is the difference in all of us that makes us unique and special. This conversation is not about hoping we understand that. Being different is awesome, it's a gift being weird is a gift, and an extension to how awesome you are. Plus, there is no such thing as weird... You are who you are, and others don't understand you "forget em" you are not here for them! Simple minded people judge others. Insecure people talk negative about others, people with low self-esteem do stupid crap like that!

You remember the "Goth" kids? I always had and still have the most respect for them! They know and understand the "Forget em" tactic. They don't acknowledge the "Cool Kids" because in their eyes that isn't what they see as cool! They don't seek your approval or acceptance. They do not bother anyone and don't need anyone to tell then what to like! Respect, respect, respect! I am not saying they are perfect because no one is, but they get it! They are cool with whomever is cool with them! They don't really care if you look or dress like them but, they appreciate when they can relate to you. I am sure someone is reading this and taking it all the wrong way... Please do yourself a favor and keep reading.

Do you love yourself?

It's a simple question...

Most people say yes, some say I think I do, and some say I dunno...

All those answers are ok. At least you are on the fence in some cases and just need to see the light. You need to "Shut up and love". Now for the people who said "Yes, they love themselves that's great for the others... Let's talk... What is it you don't love and why can't you change or fix it? Some of it is an easy fix. Some people are not happy with their weight (Exercise or eat better), some people are lonely (Go out more take risk and meet people), and some people don't really have a reason they just know they are not happy with who they are. Now please, please, PLEASE! If you have made it this far and you are saying to yourself, I hate this guy... I hate his outlook; he doesn't know what the hell he is talking about!

That is a good start!

That is awesome!

Now you are getting somewhere!

To everyone else who agrees and understands where I am coming from just sit back and enjoy the ride for the next few paragraphs. For those who don't agree, or don't like the point of view I am delivering... I say that is a good start because at least you are aware of what you do not like. (Brain explodes) In order to find what you like; you must cypher through what you don't. Remember there is no wrong or right way to love yourself. As long as you are not harming yourself and others, it's pretty much fair game! I know somethings are easier said than done. For example, exercising and eating a healthy diet... Trust me I struggled with this for a long time. But you have to Shut up and face reality... The weight isn't going anywhere, the food isn't going to cook itself. Life has it's complications but, your life doesn't have to be complicated! Get it?

- The Unicorn is a complicated fantasy animal made from "F" you and sugar!
- You are made from water (Clear)... Don't add poop you don't want.

We as people look in magazines and see people or things we like. That's cool, but don't get confused and think that you can be like them... You are better than them... You are you! If you see a model in a magazine wearing a cool jacket and you go out and by said jacket, only to find out that it doesn't look as good on you as it does on the model, you can't be mad at that! You can't feel down about it. Technically that is your own fault!

You can't love others correctly until you learn to love yourself!

Now when you look at that model on the magazine, are you taking into consideration that there was an entire team of people behind that one cover? Think about it... To make that picture on the cover of that magazine come to life that model had...

1. A makeup artist.
2. A stylist.
3. An Agent.
4. Air brushed his/her body.
5. Photographer.
6. Photoshop
7. Light Person
8. A Big Ass Fan Blowing Their hair.
9. 1 Peanut And 2 Pieces of Broccoli For Breakfast
10. Hungry

I don't know about you but, I don't have any of those things aside from "Hungry" but, then again, I am always hungry! Seriously... You are upset you don't look or can somehow look like the person that has like 50 people in a room going out of their way to make this one individual look good so you can go and buy, the product he/she is wearing!? I don't think that's fair on yourself. I don't even think it's realistic!!!! That is the point I am driving here! Living a "Real" life!

Not saying you can't compete with the model in the magazine because you can! The point is you must be real with every aspect of the situation. Being real with yourself and your surroundings is key! Do what makes you feel good, makes you feel pretty makes you feel confident! Forget everyone's opinion. The only opinion that matters is yours when it comes to how you look! That magazine isn't there for you to try to mimic the person on the cover... It is a gesture... It is someone else's opinion of what they believe looks good. Not only that, but in some situations the people behind the photo (including the model themselves) don't even like the freaking picture! They are paid to wear that nonsense; they are sponsored by someone (Company) that told them to wear that bull crap! You ever read magazines and see the section where the paparazzi caught pictures of actors, models, or musicians just walking around on a regular day or on vacation? THEY ARE NEVER WEARING THAT CRAP! They look the complete freaking opposite! Unless they are at a party or event, they -9 out of 10 times- are wearing what you are wearing in your bedroom while you were crying over their picture in the magazine.... PAJAMAS!

Amazing... They are either tired of it or don't even believe in the message they are selling you! Their job isn't always their reality. That Unicorn isn't going to go easy on you because you wear some fine designer name brand threads! You can't take any of that junk with you when you are gone! Think outside the box, be honest with yourself and your environment. I cannot stress enough that your life isn't as complicated as you make it. Life itself can be complicated but, your life doesn't have to be, and honestly probably isn't.

Do not look for approval. Be confident and real with yourself. The crazy part is that a lot of times the people we look up to or desire to be like are looking for approval from us and their atmosphere. Many times, they are so disconnected from what they believe to be cool and what actually is. Plus, what is cool to them may not be cool for everyone. I know sometimes it comes off like a broken record but, that's only because it's a true message that needs to be heard. Truth that we don't want to accept always sounds annoying.

Square Dancing In A Circle.

The art of standing out. The art of being yourself in any

atmosphere. The art of looking like a square in a circle of people that really don't matter to you or your life. The art of Standing out where others want to fit in.

<u>The art of "Forget em"</u>

They say all men are created equal... So why did she say her ex had a bigger one?

CHAPTER 7

YOUR ATMOSPHERE

(YOU'RE AT MOST FEAR)

Your Atmosphere

You are a product of your environment! Look out your window... Are there people walking around? Do they at times look like they have a destination or a goal to their day? Better yet, do they look like they are scared or hiding from something?

That last question is probably answered with "No". They don't look like they are scared or hiding... So why are you? Fear can control you, put you at a standstill or destroy you from within. Fear is probably the number one dream killer! Fear of what others may think, fear of failure, fear of not being able to do something, or... Just plain fear for no apparent reason! All those fears are understandable but not realistic! The fear you should be the most afraid of is "Not Trying At All".

They say life is short... Hmm.. is it? Or is it that we are not paying attention? If you gave attention to every single moment of your life would it seem short? You ever looked at a clock waiting for 5 minutes to past by? Seems long as hell don't it! You ever been at work and only have 30 minutes left on your shift but, those 30 minutes feel like 2 hours? Imagine, just imagine if you gave that much attention to everything you do? If you made everyday count, every hustle count, every freaking move you make count life would be a little longer! You ever looked on social media and see people doing so many things, that it makes you wonder "Where the hell do, they find the damn time to do all this stuff"? They are making every moment count! Now don't get me wrong, I am aware that a huge portion of them are just delaying pics and posting them in an order to look busy, but there is that other half... Some of them we know personally that stay on GO!

They don't allow their atmosphere to put them "At Most Fear". *(I know that sounds weird saying it but, you get the point I am making)* The Unicorn is going to go about it's business with or without you. It is going to stick it's flaming sword in the butts of who it desires daily... The question is are you going to stick around and have your ass opened in the wind waiting to see if you're next? We can all take notes from the Unicorn *(I hope by now we all know the Unicorn is "Life" I should not have to repeat this anymore cool?)* The Unicorn is PINK! Strong, doesn't give a crap about your opinion! Has rainbow wings and it's rider is gender free! It can appear as a Male or Female to the beholder! The sword it carries is bright, loud, and ready just for you! Most of all the Unicorn and it's rider make every second count! They are ready to ram your butt daily! They are ready to laugh and chuckle at your struggle and when they do, they ride off into the sunset because they can't waste time watching you even if they would love to see the outcome of what they did to you! Life (Unicorn) doesn't stop...

It's always on go and will leave you so far behind, that when you finally get the balls to do something... It may be too late!

Granted, it's never too late to start on something, but it can get to late to finish. If you are promoting something that is coming out soon and you miss your deadline... You lost your audience. If at work, you didn't meet the deadline you may lose your job or not get that bonus! Which brings us back to P.P.P. *(I'm not repeating what P.P.P. is if you were paying attention you would remember flip back to the 1st chapter or whatever if you forgot... That's that Unicorn love).*

What are you afraid of and why? Who gave you that fear? Was it you? Is it all in your head? Are you not being real with yourself? Let's say you are not going forward due to fear of death. Just as an example... Think about this... You are going to die anyway. Not saying go out there and get yourself killed. I mean if you are afraid to do something in fear of failing at it, you're not trying, YOU ALREADY FAILED AT IT! Not trying is failing! Failing is not trying! When you try and don't succeed, that is not failure that is practice, that is study, that is called "Perfecting a craft dummy". Practice makes perfect and perfect is impossible... But, perfect to your own standard is! What is perfect for you may not be perfect for the next but, it is progress non the less. The world keeps spinning, people keep evolving, changing their minds, choosing different things to do and try. That is why a real grinder, hustler doesn't understand the concept of "Perfect". The grind never stops... The hard work pays off to allow you to make it better than yesterday.

You buy a car fresh off the lot. A brand-new car never been driven... Is it perfect? Are you adding tints? Are you adding rims? Are you adding speakers? Ah well... it wasn't perfect. It was as close to perfect from the creator to sell and make money on it and next year release a better version! You need to understand the reality of the Unicorn... It's here allowing you to dwell in it's space but, that dwelling time is limited. You need to make it count! "We are not immortal". We are not a Rolex watch where we can stop ticking and keep going. Once we stop ticking... This is over! In my opinion that is what we should really fear! Fear that when you look back at your life you did nothing but, ducked down from the Unicorn every time it came by your neighborhood. This is not to inspire you... If inspiration is what you think you have been reading this entire time, then you must be mistaken!

This is reality... Everyone's reality is that we all have one major thing in common, we are not immortal... We are on borrowed time... We have nothing to fear but, fear itself. You know what? That fear you are afraid of, Is you!

It's not easy to break a routine. Fear is a routine. Once you face it and overcome it, the routine is broken. The fear is eliminated. Square dancing in a circle requires balance... We must be careful where we step and always pay attention to our surroundings. The metaphor behind square dancing a circle is Standing out where everyone is fitting in. Don't allow your atmosphere to put you at your most fear. You will never know if the water is cold if you don't at least stick a toe in. Therefore, the moral to the story here is go at your own pace but have a pace. Standing still in fear of what will happen is not a pace. The world around you could be crumbling but, you can make it through the chaos if you tread carefully. Life is a marathon not a 100 MPH race. The finish line is nowhere in sight. Even the most successful in this world pass and still feel like there is so much more they could have done! As long as we can walk this earth, we will always feel the need to explore, to expand, and to create.

A famous movie once said, "Take risk, you don't want to die without any scars".

While some of you don't like the reality of death being brought up so many times, others grasp the concept of it. They grip the Unicorns balls as hard as they can and ride it to the next level! Wake up, snap out of it. Your greatness is distracted by your atmosphere.

Success is not a job, position, or title. Success is you! You take who you are and apply success to it. If you get a promotion the success is not the promotion. The success is you and you apply success to the promotion. That is why you were chosen to have bigger challenges than most. That is why it is difficult for you to break free of the fear routine....

You are given a circle platform, with square dancing skills from the beginning.

Master that and you will have balance.

You will overcome fear. After that?

There is no more "At Most Fear" (Atmosphere)... You are At Your Most in This Sphere.

Sphere = Earth.

People always want space... But no one wants to be an Astronaut.

CHAPTER 8

UNICORNS AND DOG POOP

(REALITY VS FANTASY)

UNICORNS AND DOG SHIT

It's Saturday morning you wake up slide into your slippers and head to the bathroom. You don't have to go to work today and your Wife/Husband actually had to work today. The kids are at their Grandparents house. You are home alone... The king/Queen has the kingdom to themselves.

You take a deep breath (AAAHHHhhhhhhh!!!) You look in the mirror and see the toilet behind you. Clean, shiny, white and the seat is down. It's calling you... You are in no rush so before you brush your teeth you take a long relaxing dump, while looking through your social media outlets. The world is in chaos, everyone is losing their minds and your favorite artist just announced they will no longer be making music. That sucks but, you are so relaxed and don't give a crap! You wipe your butt, don't even flush cause again this morning "You don't give a crap". You brush your teeth, go downstairs, and feed your dog/cat. Your partner made coffee so it's freshly brewed and ready. You are hungry but, not starving so you pop in something simple like waffles into the toaster. "Pop"... They eject and you snatch it up with your coffee and walk out to your well-groomed back yard. Your cell phone rings and it's your boss telling you he recognizes the hard work you have been doing and gives you a raise just cause! He tells you take tomorrow off with pay and you put the phone down, take a smooth sip of coffee and a deep breath along with it! (AAAAAAAHHHHHHH!!!)

You open your eyes after your deep inhale and before you can exhale, a beautiful Unicorn appears from behind the trees... Long Rainbow hair, tall stallion strong! Wings that span across your back yard and a horn that looks like king Arthur's sword. You smile and it smiles back and bends over and takes a huge, wet, slimy "Dog poop" on your roses. It attempts to cover the dog poop with it's hooves but, ends up chucking chunks of it at your face and into your coffee. It turns around looks at you and spreads it's wings and in one big push it swoops into the sky and takes off breaking the sound barrier and splashing the crappy hot coffee all over your chest! It burns so much that you jump up only to realize you fell asleep during your lunch break at work. Your late returning and you actually knocked over the coffee into your lap. Then when things couldn't get any worst... Your Boss walks in and says, "I want to see you in my office."

<u>This fool!.</u>

The reality is everything in the dream up until the Unicorn defecating over your roses can exist. The fantasy part is believing it will happen without change. Not change in your character, clothing, or personality, but change in your outlook and drive. The system of life is designed by a higher power, by forces and reasons we are not yet ready to comprehend. Hence, the forever on going question... What is the meaning of life? Well while others search for answers, they will not get anytime soon... Why not instead of asking what is the meaning of life, give your life meaning? (Head explodes)

Unicorns love marathons and we are all in it. Every single one of us are in it together. The crazy part is, even though we are all together we live inside this fantasy that we are all in competition with each other. Some of us are just jogging and daydreaming, others jogging in place, and others are sitting down with the illusion and fantasy that it will get better. That water will fall from the sky and quench their thirst for a better tomorrow. While they sit there waiting, here comes the good old Unicorn with fire on his dick this time. Ready to double charge you for a free Sunday.

Reality and fantasy go hand and hand. In it's on way reality can infuse a fantasy into existence. The trick is to know how to manipulate the system. We all can't have the Unicorns just drop us off a plate of cash and some tickets to a free and better tomorrow. Yes, some people are privileged enough to be born into the "silver spoon in their mouth" world. While others (Like myself) are born into the "wooden spoon that give you splinters on your lip's" world. We could blame it on our parents, I guess. It would be easier to say "Mom, Dad... Why you fools broke? Why the hell does this damn spoon have so many splinters and smell like we scoop raisins out of a camel's butt with it?"

Then what?

Complain some more?

Go to work with an attitude?

Be mad at the Unicorns?

Seek attention from others by saying, "nothing's wrong" when they ask you what's wrong, only to get mad when they say "Ok" and walk off?

Get real!

There are some people in situations where they lose a loved one… Mom, dad, etc.… and they find a way to move on. Then you have those same people lose a cat or a dog and are devastated. They are ready to give up on life! Trust me when I say I get it. We are attached to what we are attached to. Maybe more of a connection was made between you and the dog than the connection between you and your mother. The outcome is still the same. You're in pain and it hurts so much that you want to rip your heart out and throw it in the ocean! The process is the same (One is more expensive than the other) you must bury them or burn them to ashes and find a way to cope and move on.

That's the reality…

The fantasy is walking around angry. Blaming others and seeking attention from people who don't even know what's wrong. Pain and loss of someone is hard for anyone. For some, to get over it is easier for them, tough for others, and impossible for few. That's where the fantasy kicks in and we ourselves become the Unicorn. (Trust me that's not a good thing). Becoming the Unicorn is when you lose total control. You lose yourself in the pain. You get lost in the forest of regret and (could've, would've, should've) …. Then you retaliate on life.

No one understands you; no one has gone through the pain you are going through. Everyone is stupid and full of crap. No one cares about you and they are all about themselves! The list goes on and on! Even though many will not like this part… That is the "Fantasy".

The reality is many have gone through what you are going through, and many have gone through worst. Many understand you and can relate to your pain. Many are looking at you like you are lost, stupid, full of crap and lost a grip with reality. They see you slipping, and many are trying to help. You're just too deep in your fantasy of anger that you can't see that.

The same treatment applies to relationships, jobs, friends, and finances. When we lose any of these things, we tend to lose control and only a few can handle the drastic lost and rebuild. Now don't get me wrong, I am not saying "Oh, you lost your mother, that was a week ago, get over it." No… That is not the case I am building here. I am saying time heals all wounds… But you are in a fantasy world if you keep picking at it. If you don't face it head on and realize your position and let the cut heal. It is ok to be mad, it is ok to be sad, angry, and upset plus drastically hurt! What is not ok is losing yourself in the process.

If we lose control who watches those depending on us? The kids, The dog etc…. Who watches them? (If they are in the picture) Not only that what about the people that depend on you? Friends, family members, they are in pain for the same reason. The Unicorns that run the circle of life do not provide the dog poop… We do. WE ARE NOT IMMORTAL. We are strong but fragile. Smart but, weak minded at times. The ones we lose don't want us to lose ourselves as well. They want us to rise up and prosper. Carry their legacy to the next level so the same can be done for you. Tick Tock is reality… Pausing the clock is fantasy.

I haven't said this in a while "Love It".

The game gets better as you master each challenge.

The game gets better when you level up!

The game gets better when you evolve.

You don't have to necessarily love the game, but you can love who you are in the game. You can love your avatar that was given to you in the game. Take care of it, treat it as if it were yours because when the time runs out, you may never see it again. You must upgrade it, tune it up, wash it, nurture it.

Look around the room and ask yourself... Who can give you what you want?

Only You can!

Let's talk Less talk... (Read that again LOL)

It's funny to say Let's talk about talking less. It's an awesome contradiction. What is really means is let's talk more about the work and push and less about the talking it up part. Now yes, they say speak things into existence... I swear a person that lives in a fantasy world said that to me once. He had me there speaking a million bucks into existence, the only million that took place was the millions of seconds and minutes nothing happened! People take phrases and take them "too many times" as what they say versus what they are saying. "Speak things into existence" isn't say it till it happens. That's equivalent to that other phrase "Fake it till you make it" Geez! Who came up with that abomination!?

Ok... People always speak about being real and how they want you to be real around them and only the real, real, real! So, you're going to act fake and lie to my face about what you have, do, and are, until one day it's actually real?

So, our friendship was based on a lie this entire time! If you fake it too long and too much you will master the art of lies and being fake so much that when you finally "Make it", you will be faker than you were before! Because if acting like you had "this and that" had you acting the way you were acting, when it becomes reality you will be "Dog poop".

When you are fake (Dog poop fantasy) for so long, you forget how to be real (Unicorn). Not only that, have you ever heard the phrase "Real recognize real". You need to ask yourself... Are your friends real? Are the people around you that you know and trust real? Because if they were... Do they recognize you? (Head Explosion)

Let's get back to speaking things into existence and taking action. Taking action and speaking things into existence is the same thing with different clothing on. You speak things into your mind, see it in your head, visualize it! Breathe it in and almost taste it! Then once you are there, that feeling of being so close... Creates the drive which makes you take action.

Now you are a Unicorn who can identify Dog poop!

If they piss on your face & say it's raining... They must drink a lot of water!

Because you can smell pee... It's kind of salty too!

CHAPTER 9

WE ARE NOT IMMORTAL

(GET OVER THAT CRAP OR LET IT GO)

WE ARE NOT IMMORTAL

That title kind of speaks for itself. We have been stating that through the previous chapters.

Heart break

Holding grudges

Having too much pride

Apologizing

Forgiveness

Remorse

Trapped

Being honest with yourself

Fear

Procrastination

Pain

Suffering

Being Honest to others

Acceptance

Success

Failure

Sadness

Happiness

Joy

Hate

The electric bill

Mowing the freaking lawn... Wait what?

Aside from the last two the rest of the things mentioned on this list falls under the guidelines of "We are not immortal". We get to complacent with the idea of putting things off as if we are here until the end of time.

Picture if you will, that you are upset with your sister/ brother for whatever reason! Now a few days pass by and you still are holding on to whatever it is. Then a month, then a year or two passes by. We get so comfortable at the idea of not speaking until we are ready, or we just put it off and charge it to "Out of sight out of mind". Then by the time you come to realize it has been 4 years and you both just got comfortable with the idea of not addressing it. Then one day you get the phone call that your sibling has passed away.

Here we go with the nonsense.

This is what your sound like now...

I should have called them.

I cannot believe their gone!

I hope they knew I loved them more than anything.

I should have this...

I should have that...

You should have...

Just...

Shut up & Love!

Now here we go with the water works... You need to take a chapter out of "We are not Immortal". Handle that Stupid stuff now. Too many times we are faced with situations that could have easily been handled. Too many times we are in a relationship we don't like or love anymore.

Heart Break!

Picture this... You get dumped or cheated on by your significant other, now you are understandably hurt beyond belief. You can't believe what has happened and you honestly didn't see this day coming. You try calling back, sending text messages, emails the works. He/She never responds but, one day finally does and all they say to you is "Please leave me alone" ....OUCH!

How long is it ok to mourn over this situation in your opinion? I guess it depends on the person it happened to, how long they were together and how deep into the relationship they were. Either way you reach a limit where you have to move on! See, while you're there suffering, hurt, ignoring life, and allowing yourself to fall deeper. Your significant other has moved on and has a new boy/girlfriend getting their back blown out, rode on, and steam rolled over deep/hard and forgot you possibly existed. It doesn't matter what the breakup was over, cheated or just a breakup, you reach a point where you have to allow the pain to take it's course and move on.

Now when you move on, you have to collect yourself and make sure you don't bring the pain with you to the next relationship. You know what they call that? '

Damaged goods!

Remember "We are not immortal"

You can't expect every single person you meet and attempt to have a new relationship with to attend to your already old self "closed but you keep opening them back up" wounds! That new person you met has nothing to do with your past, they weren't there and it's not their responsibility to cure, help, or fix your broken self. That is up you.

You have to "Shut upand "LOVE" yourself 1st before you move on to another.

Holding on to pain isn't good for the soul. Holding grudges

with people you know deep inside you miss and love like crazy isn't going to do you any good. If you know deep inside there is something to rekindle then make the call, send the text or email. Now don't get it twisted ... I am referring to situations like fall outs with your parents, friends, family members, etc.... I don't mean ex boy/girlfriends.

We are not immortal!

Forgiveness is important... Especially self-forgiveness! Remember you have to...

Shut up "LOVE" yourself! Love yourself enough to forgive yourself. Pain runs deep and can pull you into a dark place that doesn't allow you to come back. Sometimes you come back as something else because you allow yourself to fall to deep! It's a scary place because you can actually reach a point of no return. You lose friends, you lose family, you lose yourself, and you lose time! We are not immortal! If we lose time, we lose it all. Time can heal but, it can also steal!

Time can heal and it can steal.

Think about it.

It's scary!

We are not immortal....

Forgive yourself, let go, allow yourself to heal and live love, love life!

CHAPTER 10

YOU'RE ALIVE, BUT ARE YOU LIVING?

(DO YOU UNDERSTAND YET?)

YOU'RE ALIVE BUT, ARE YOU LIVING?

Ok so here we are... How do you feel? I don't expect you to lift your head out of the pages and say, "Yeah man I get it to hell with that Unicorn and that idiot riding it to". Ha! Ha! No... Now don't get me wrong, if that's how you feel Congratulations, you've officially graduated from kiss my behind academy!

On a serious note... You're Alive but, Are You Living? should be a way of life to many. It's not about being cold hearted or thick skinned. It is not about "not giving a freak" or anything like that. It is honestly about looking forward, looking towards tomorrow, and realizing how special you are. Realize how important your life is and don't waste it on subjects that don't matter. Imagine if the world understood this concept! Imagine if people in power could follow this idea! Picture people not getting mad enough to go out and kill someone. Picture people looking at themselves in the mirror and realizing how they can change things around, love themselves, love their friends, family, strangers, and their atmosphere.

Now when we say love others... We mean in the sense of peace to everyone. The topics we have addressed are also for people to understand that the Unicorns are not here to play! The Unicorns create chaos at times, we are their entertainment... if we were a movie and the Unicorns were watching us on the big screen, some of the crap we go through is funny. The Unicorns been running the game of life before you got here, while you were here, and they will be running it decades after you leave!

The game we are involved in didn't come with an instruction manual. No guidance, aside from trial and error. Our parents learned it from their parents added some spice and passed it on as much as they could to us, and we must do the same. We woke up and the world kept spinning and if you take into consideration how huge the world is a lot can happen while you sleep. It's a sad, hard, and scary place if you focus your attention on everything happening around the world.

The world itself is in pain.

If tomorrow you won a million dollars your perspective on life would change dramatically!

Why?

Because of the money?

Or because the money increased your confidence?

Now you want to love yourself huh? Don't allow this to happen to you... Shut up and love today! Take a new outlook on life. Realize how important you are, how much you can do if you make every moment count. Pain is going to come. Problems are always going to spawn it's self out of thin air and beat up someone's day. You may be crossing paths with that person and your day may get altered but if you tread carefully you can avoid it. You could handle your day correctly by playing the game and making sure you don't lose or get slowed down.

It's almost as if the Unicorns want us to hate ourselves; they want us to self-destruct; they want us to be reckless and chaotic. It is easier to destroy than it is to create.... It is human nature to destroy... Hate is easy to come across. You can find it anywhere. Wars start from love and end up in hate... How? People are speaking to loud at times and do not listen to each other... They fight and never allow themselves to take a step back and say...

We are not immortal.

Maybe I should just "Live and not just be Alive"!

What Goes Around Comes Around...

Ask Yourself, Are You Coming Or Going?

CESSATION

(WE ABOUT TO RIDE THE UNICORN HOME)

CESSATION

I didn't want to do this in the beginning because I felt I would be putting a somewhat bias opinion on your point of view. I wanted you to read this and take a lot or at least a good portion that will help you tomorrow and going forward.

What inspired "You're Alive but, Are You Living?"

Make a "really long" story short, life inspired it. As I stated in the beginning of the book. My mother died from Cancer. She was an amazing woman and strong (Who doesn't say that about their mother?) The one thing that always intrigued me about her was her humor. She joked and laughed all the way to the grave! My mother's last words to me while she was extremely sick were...

"Life is one big joke... Waiting to be laughed at".

At the time I had no clue what the hell she was talking about. I just smiled and cried. She giggled and I remember she started coughing and that was the last time I heard her voice. As time went by and it became a little easier for me to think of her and not break down, I started looking back at a lot of situations and scenarios in my life. If my life was being viewed through a lens onto a movie theater screen.... My life would be a pretty funny twisted story to watch! It's like damn... How much pain are they going to put this guy through before he snaps? I would watch the movie in fear that he was going to lose total control and kill somebody or everybody!

The more I looked back and thought about it, not in pain, just honestly thinking back and replaying life in my head... I started laughing and realized something. Geez man! My life really isn't as complicated as I thought it was, life around me is! Everything going wrong, bad or as some say left! All of it was out of my control.

My Brother being shot in front of me and killed.

My Dad being murdered after he won the lottery.

My Mother dying of cancer.

Divorce

Best friend dying in a car crash.

Struggles to see my kids.

Being Homeless for 4 months.

Getting arrested and put in holding for being at the wrong place at the wrong time. (No Charges, I just wanted to throw that in there I am not A Gangsta! LOL)

Betrayed by a few friends and almost being killed by them twice.

I could go on with more but, those are the highlights LOL. As I looked back at all of it and realized I haven't been broken down, I am not damaged goods. Life (The Freaking Unicorns) are always messing around and causing chaos around us. We are all in this together but, struggling individually. I realized I was given a gift and a curse. The gift and the curse of understanding my emotions connected to life and the way the Unicorns can affect us. I've seen my mother do everything she could to balance her world. Struggled half her life to finally reach the top and buy a big house…... She died before she could enjoy it.

My dad was something else. Always trying to find a short cut through life and he found one when he won the lottery…. Then was killed… Talk about a short cut huh?

My Brother was a church going, God fearing man! Didn't curse and was very well respected by everyone. Body builder and all-around best friend and hated violence and was killed by random gun fire!

That's when it hit me! WHOA…. We are not immortal. We don't know when we are going to clock out.

The Dream…

That same night I had a dream that I was in the woods running and I couldn't see what I was running from! I just knew it was fast and trying to end me! I ran, jumped, and dived through the woods and thought I lost it! It was bright as hell outside… The sun was shining, and the rivers were flowing…

Then it happened...

The sun just left... it was pitch black... The moon was nowhere to be found! The river went dry and the woods got extremely quiet! I couldn't even see my hands in front of my face. It felt like I went blind and deaf at the same time... I didn't know what came over me but, I clenched my fist really hard opened my eyes and yelled at the top of my lungs! Just a yell, no words just....

AAAAAARRRRGGGGGGHHHHHHHH!!!!!!!!!!!!!!!!!!!!!!!!!!!!!!!!!!!!!

Then that's when it appeared! Light shining from the darkness. It got closer and closer, I could hear the footsteps getting closer and my legs were frozen in fear! Then I saw it!

A Pink Unicorn, Long rainbow hair, Beautiful tail, gold hooves... With an elegant sexy "thick in all the right places" Goddess riding on top of the Unicorn holding a sword covered in fire! I thought it was there to save me from the darkness... No... She looked at me and said, "Run bitch... Entertain me"!

I woke up so enlightened with this extreme sense of bravery. It was that night I realized so many things... We are Not immortal... We are not here forever... We are here on borrowed time... We have to make every day count... We need to stop complaining...

We Need to "Live Life and not Just be ALIVE"

Raxiel Liz
@Raxiel_Liz

Other projects
I didn't know my daughter was a ninja (Book)
F*CK 2020 – 2021 JOURNAL (Journal)
I'm not weird, deep inside I'm a DRAGON (Journal)
Mistakes and Monster (Script ebook)
Director's Cut (Script ebook)
Mistakes and Monsters (Movie)
Raxiel Sinz (Music on all digital platforms)
We Alive and Living (YouTube Channel)

Make sure to look into these for more projects from Raxiel Liz

Love

YOU'RE ALIVE BUT, ARE YOU LIVING?

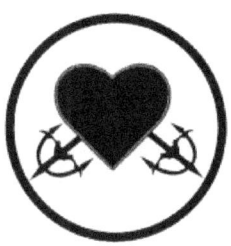

The Unicorns Are Always Plotting

I am going to leave a few pages blank so you can jot down some ideas, drawings doodles or carry like a small journal so this book isn't just a book you throw on the shelves after you're done reading it.

Enjoy

And

Thank you!

RAXIELLIZ